Slow Cooker Breakfast Delights

Tasty and delicious Breakfast & Brunch

to Start Your Day

Donna Conway

implied. readers acknowledge that the author is not engaging in the rendering of legal, financial, medical or professional advice. the content within this book has been derived from various sources. please consult a licensed professional before attempting any techniques outlined in this book.

by reading this document, the reader agrees that under no circumstances is the author responsible for any losses, direct or indirect, which are incurred as a result of the use of information contained within this document, including, but not limited to, — errors, omissions, or inaccuracies.

Table of Contents

Different Chicken Dip

Preparation time: 10 minutes

Cooking time: 3 hours and 30 minutes

Servings: 4 people

Ingredients:

- 1 yellow onion, chopped

- 2 teaspoons olive oil

- 1 red bell pepper, chopped

- 3 cups rotisserie chicken, cooked and shredded

- 12 oz. coconut cream

- ½ cup chili sauce

- 2 tablespoons chives, chopped

Directions:

1. Heat-up a pan with the oil over medium-high heat, add the onion, stir, cook for 5 minutes and transfer to your slow cooker.

2. Add bell pepper, cream, chicken, chili sauce, chives, toss, cover, cook on low for 3 hours and 30 minutes, divide into bowls and serve as a party dip. Enjoy!

Nutrition:

Calories: 251

Fat: 5g

Carbs: 17g

Protein: 18g

Carrot Dip

Preparation time: 10 minutes

Cooking time: 5 hours

Servings: 4

Ingredients:

- 2-pound carrots, peeled and chopped

- ¼ cup olive oil

- 2 teaspoons cumin, ground

- A pinch of salt and black pepper

- 4 garlic cloves, minced

- ½ cup veggie stock

Directions:

1. Grease your slow cooker with half of the oil, add carrots, cumin, salt, pepper, garlic, and stock, toss,

cover, cook on low for 5 hours, transfer to your blender, add the rest of the oil, pulse well, divide into bowls and serve. Enjoy!

Nutrition:

Calories: 211

Fat: 6g

Carbs: 13g

Protein: 7g

Pepperoni Dip

Preparation time: 10 minutes

Cooking time: 1 hour

Servings: 4 people

Ingredients:

- 13 oz. coconut cream
- 8 oz. pepperoni, sliced
- A pinch of black pepper

Directions:

1. In your slow cooker, combine the cream with the pepperoni and black pepper, cover, cook on low for 1 hour, stir, divide into bowls and serve. Enjoy!

Nutrition: Calories: 231, Fat: 4g, Carbs: 16g, Protein: 11g

Eggplant Spread

Preparation time: 10 minutes

Cooking time: 1 hour and 30 minutes

Servings: 4 people

Ingredients:

- 2 pounds eggplants, peeled and cubed
- 1 tablespoon sesame paste
- 3 tablespoons lemon juice
- 1 garlic clove, minced
- ¼ teaspoon liquid smoke
- ½ teaspoon olive oil
- Handful parsley, chopped

Directions:

1. In your slow cooker, combine the eggplants with the sesame paste, lemon juice, garlic, liquid smoke, oil,

parsley, toss, cover, cook on high for 1 hour and 30 minutes, pulse using an immersion blender, and serve. Enjoy!

Nutrition:

Calories: 211

Fat: 4g

Carbs: 15g

Protein: 7g

Jalapeno Poppers

Preparation time: 10 minutes

Cooking time: 3 hours

Servings: 4 people

Ingredients:

- ½ pound chorizo, chopped
- 10 jalapenos, tops cut off and deseeded
- 1 small white onion, chopped
- ½ pound beef, ground
- ¼ teaspoon garlic powder
- 1 tablespoon maple syrup
- 1 tablespoon mustard
- 1/3 cup water

Directions:

1. Mix the beef with chorizo, garlic powder, and onion in a bowl. Stuff your jalapenos with the mix and put them in your slow cooker.

2. Put the water, cover, and cook on high within 3 hours. Move the jalapeno poppers to a lined baking sheet. In a bowl, mix maple syrup with mustard and whisk well.

3. Brush poppers with this mix, introduce in the preheated broiler and cook for 10 minutes. Arrange on a platter and serve. Enjoy!

Nutrition:

Calories: 200

Fat: 2g

Carbs: 8g

Protein: 3g

Fish Sticks

Preparation time: 10 minutes

Cooking time: 2 hours

Servings: 4 people

Ingredients:

- 2 eggs, whisked

- 1-pound cod fillets, cut into medium strips

- 1 and ½ cups almond flour

- A pinch of sea salt

- Black pepper to the taste

- ½ cup tapioca flour

- ¼ teaspoon paprika

- Cooking spray

Directions:

1. In a bowl, mix almond flour, salt, pepper, tapioca, and paprika and stir. Put the eggs in another bowl.

Dip fish sticks in the eggs and then dredge in the flour mix.

2. Spray your slow cooker with cooking spray and arrange fish sticks in it—cover and cook on high within 2 hours. Arrange on a platter and serve. Enjoy!

Nutrition:

Calories: 200

Fat: 2g

Carbs: 7g

Protein: 12g

Spicy Pecans

Preparation time: 10 minutes

Cooking time: 2 hours and 15 minutes

Servings: 4 people

Ingredients:

- 1-pound pecans halved
- 2 tablespoons olive oil
- 1 teaspoon basil, dried
- 1 tablespoon chili powder
- 1 teaspoon oregano, dried
- ¼ teaspoon garlic powder
- 1 teaspoon thyme, dried
- ½ teaspoon onion powder
- A pinch of cayenne pepper

Directions:

1. In your slow cooker, mix pecans with oil, basil, chili powder, oregano, garlic powder, onion powder, thyme, and cayenne and toss to coat.

2. Cover and cook on high within 15 minutes. Switch slow cooker to low and cook for 2 hours. Serve as a snack. Enjoy!

Nutrition:

Calories: 78

Fat: 3g

Carbs: 9g

Protein: 2g

Sausage Appetizer

Preparation time: 10 minutes

Cooking time: 2 hours

Servings: 15 sausages

Ingredients:

- 2 pounds sausages, sliced
- 18 oz. unsweetened apple jelly
- 9 oz. Dijon mustard

Directions:

1. Place sausage slices in your slow cooker, add apple jelly and mustard and toss to coat well. Cover and cook on low within 2 hours, stirring every 20 minutes. Arrange sausage slices on a platter and serve as an appetizer. Enjoy!

Nutrition: Calories: 140, Fat: 3g, Carbs: 9g, Protein: 10g

Asparagus Spread

Preparation time: 10 minutes

Cooking time: 2 hours and 30 minutes

Servings: 4 people

Ingredients:

- 1 bunch asparagus, roughly chopped
- 4 garlic cloves, minced
- 5 oz. coconut cream
- ½ teaspoon garlic powder
- ½ teaspoon red pepper flakes
- ¼ teaspoon onion powder
- ¼ teaspoon paprika
- 6 oz. baby spinach
- 2 teaspoons olive oil
- ½ cup veggie stock

Directions:

1. In your slow cooker, combine the asparagus with the garlic, cream, garlic powder, pepper flakes, onion powder, paprika, spinach, stock, and oil, toss, cover, cook on low for 2 hours and 30 minutes, pulse using an immersion blender and serve. Enjoy!

Nutrition:

Calories: 221

Fat: 4g

Carbs: 16g

Protein: 8g

Broccoli Dip

Preparation time: 10 minutes

Cooking time: 2 hours

Servings: 4 people

Ingredients:

- 1 yellow onion, chopped
- 6 bacon slices, cooked and chopped
- 2 garlic cloves, minced
- ¼ teaspoon red pepper flakes, crushed
- 4 cups broccoli florets, chopped
- 8 oz. coconut cream
- 1 tablespoon scallions, chopped
- ½ cup avocado mayonnaise
- ½ cup of coconut milk
- A pinch of salt and black pepper

Directions:

1. In your slow cooker, combine the onion with the bacon, garlic, pepper flakes, broccoli, cream, scallions, mayo, milk, salt and pepper, stir, cover, cook on low for 2 hours, stir again really well, divide into bowls and serve. Enjoy!

Nutrition:

Calories: 261

Fat: 11g

Carbs: 8g

Protein: 12g

Crab and Onion Dip

Preparation time: 10 minutes

Cooking time: 4 hours

Servings: 4 people

Ingredients:

- 24 oz. coconut cream
- 12 oz. canned crabmeat, drained
- ¼ cup of coconut milk
- 4 green onions, chopped
- 2 teaspoons horseradish, prepared
- A pinch of salt and black pepper

Directions:

1. In your slow cooker, combine the cream with the crabmeat, milk, onions, salt, pepper, and

horseradish, stir, cover, cook on low for 4 hours, divide into bowls and serve. Enjoy!

Nutrition:

Calories: 167

Fat: 8g

Carbs: 2g

Protein: 7g

Spinach and Bacon Dip

Preparation time: 10 minutes

Cooking time: 2 hours

Servings: 4 people

Ingredients:

- 16 oz. coconut cream
- 1 cup of coconut milk
- 15 oz. canned artichokes, drained and chopped
- 10 oz. spinach, chopped
- 2 tomatoes, chopped
- ½ cup bacon, cooked and crumbled
- 4 green onions, chopped

Directions:

1. In your slow cooker, combine the cream with coconut milk, spinach, artichokes, tomatoes, and green

onions, stir, cover, cook on low for 2 hours, divide

into bowls, sprinkle bacon on top, and serve. Enjoy!

Nutrition:

Calories: 200

Fat: 6g

Carbs: 9g

Protein: 6g

Bean Pesto Dip

Preparation time: 15 minutes

Cooking time: 6 hours

Servings: 4 people

Ingredients:

- 10 oz. refried beans
- 1 tbsp pesto sauce
- 1 tsp salt
- 7 oz. Cheddar cheese, shredded
- 1 tsp paprika
- 1 cup of salsa
- 4 tbsp sour cream
- 2-oz. cream cheese
- 1 tsp dried dill

Directions:

1. Mix pesto with salt, salsa, sour cream, dill, beans, cheese, paprika, and cream cheese in the slow cooker.

2. Put the cooker's lid on and set the cooking time to 6 hours on low. Blend the mixture using a hand blender. Serve fresh.

Nutrition:

Calories: 102

Fat: 6.3g

Carbs: 7.43g

Protein: 5g

Cheesy Chili Pepper Dip

Preparation time: 15 minutes

Cooking time: 9 hours

Servings: 4 people

Ingredients:

- 4 chili pepper, sliced and deseeded
- 7 oz. Monterey cheese
- 3 tbsp cream cheese
- 1 tbsp onion powder
- 3 tbsp dried dill
- 3 oz. butter
- 1 tbsp cornstarch
- 1 tbsp flour
- ¼ tsp salt

Directions:

1. Add chili peppers to a blender and add salt, butter, onion powder, and dill. Blend the chili peppers well, then transfer to the slow cooker.

2. Stir in flour, cornstarch, cream cheese, and Monterey cheese. Put the cooker's lid on and set the cooking time to 6 hours on low. Serve.

Nutrition:

Calories: 212

Fat: 18.2g

Carbs: 6.06g

Protein: 8g

Creamy Mushroom Spread

Preparation time: 15 minutes

Cooking time: 4 hours

Servings: 2 people

Ingredients:

- 1-pound mushrooms, sliced

- 3 garlic cloves, minced

- 1 cup heavy cream

- 2 teaspoons smoked paprika

- Salt and black pepper to the taste

- 2 tablespoons parsley, chopped

Directions:

1. In your slow cooker, mix the mushrooms with the garlic and the other ingredients, whisk, cook on low

within 4 hours. Whisk, divide into bowls, and serve as a party spread.

Nutrition:

Calories: 300,

Fat: 6g,

Carbs: 16g,

Protein: 6

Pork Tostadas

Preparation time: 15 minutes

Cooking time: 4 hours

Servings: 4 people

Ingredients:

- 4 lbs. pork shoulder, boneless and cubed
- Salt and black pepper to the taste
- 2 cups coca cola
- 1/3 cup brown sugar
- ½ cup hot sauce
- 2 tsp chili powder
- 2 tbsp tomato paste
- ¼ tsp cumin, ground
- 1 cup enchilada sauce
- Corn tortillas, toasted for a few minutes in the oven

- Mexican cheese, shredded for serving

- 4 shredded lettuce leaves, for serving

- Salsa

- Guacamole for serving

Directions:

1. Add cup coke, salsa, sugar, chili powder, cumin, pork, hot sauce, and tomato paste to the slow cooker. Put the cooker's lid on and set the cooking time to 4 hours on low.

2. Drain the cooked pork and shred it finely. Mix well the shredded pork with enchilada sauce and remaining coke.

3. Divide the pork into the tortillas and top it with lettuce leaves, guacamole, and Mexican cheese. Serve.

Nutrition:

Calories: 162, Fat: 3g, Carbs: 12g, Protein: 5g

BBQ Chicken Dip

Preparation time: 15 minutes

Cooking time: 1 hour and 30 minutes

Servings: 4 people

Ingredients:

- 1 and ½ cups BBQ sauce

- 1 small red onion, chopped

- 24 oz. cream cheese, cubed

- 2 cups rotisserie chicken, shredded

- 3 bacon slices, cooked and crumbled

- 1 plum tomato, chopped

- ½ cup cheddar cheese, shredded

- 1 tablespoon green onions, chopped

Directions:

1. In your slow cooker, mix BBQ sauce with onion, cream cheese, rotisserie chicken, bacon, tomato,

cheddar, and green onions, stir, cover, and cook on low for 1 hour and 30 minutes. Divide into bowls and serve.

Nutrition:

Calories: 251

Fat: 4g

Carbs: 10g

Protein: 4g

Lemon Shrimp Dip

Preparation time: 15 minutes

Cooking time: 2 hours

Servings: 2 people

Ingredients:

- 3 oz. cream cheese, soft
- ½ cup heavy cream
- 1-pound shrimp, peeled, deveined, and chopped
- ½ tablespoon balsamic vinegar
- 2 tablespoons mayonnaise
- ½ tablespoon lemon juice
- A pinch of salt and black pepper
- 2 oz. mozzarella, shredded
- 1 tablespoon parsley, chopped

Directions:

1. In your slow cooker, mix the cream cheese with the shrimp, heavy cream, and the other ingredients, whisk, put the lid on and cook on low for 2 hours. Divide into bowls and serve.

Nutrition:

Calories: 342

Fat: 4g

Carbs: 7g

Protein: 10g

Zucchini Sticks

Preparation time: 15 minutes

Cooking time: 2 hours

Servings: 13 sticks

Ingredients:

- 9 oz. green zucchini, cut into thick sticks

- 4 oz. Parmesan, grated

- 1 egg

- 1 tsp salt

- 1 tsp ground white pepper

- 1 tsp olive oil

- 2 tbsp milk

Directions:

1. Grease the base of your slow cooker with olive oil. Whisk egg with milk, white pepper, and salt in a bowl.

2. Dip the prepared zucchini sticks in the egg mixture, then place them in the slow cooker. Put the cooker's lid on and set the cooking time to 2 hours on high.

3. Spread the cheese over the zucchini sticks evenly. Put the cooker's lid on and set the cooking time to 2 hours on high. Serve.

Nutrition:

Calories: 51

Fat: 1.7g

Carbs: 4.62g

Protein: 5g

Chicken Cordon Bleu Dip

Preparation time: 15 minutes

Cooking time: 1 hour & 30 minutes

Servings: 4 people

Ingredients:

- 16 oz. cream cheese

- 2 chicken breasts, baked and shredded

- 1 cup cheddar cheese, shredded

- 1 cup Swiss cheese, shredded

- 3 garlic cloves, minced

- 6 oz. ham, chopped

- 2 tablespoons green onions

- Salt and black pepper to the taste

Directions:

1. In your slow cooker, mix cream cheese with chicken, cheddar cheese, Swiss cheese, garlic, ham, green

onions, salt, and pepper, stir, cover, and cook on low for 1 hour and 30 minutes. Serve.

Nutrition:

Calories: 243

Fat: 5g

Carbs: 15g

Protein: 3g

Eggplant Zucchini Dip

Preparation time: 15 minutes

Cooking time: 4 hours & 5 minutes

Servings: 4 people

Ingredients:

- 1 eggplant
- 1 zucchini, chopped
- 2 tbsp olive oil
- 2 tbsp balsamic vinegar
- 1 tbsp parsley, chopped
- 1 yellow onion, chopped
- 1 celery stick, chopped
- 1 tomato, chopped
- 2 tbsp tomato paste
- 1 and ½ tsp garlic, minced

- A pinch of sea salt

- Black pepper to the taste

Directions:

1. Rub the eggplant with cooking oil and grill it for 5 minutes per side on a preheated grill. Chop the grilled eggplant and transfer it to the slow cooker.

2. Add tomato, parsley, and all other ingredients to the cooker. Put the cooker's lid on and set the cooking time to 4 hours on high. Serve.

Nutrition:

Calories: 110

Fat: 1g

Carbs: 7g

Protein: 5g

Calamari Rings Bowls

Preparation time: 15 minutes

Cooking time: 6 hours

Servings: 2 people

Ingredients:

- ½ pound calamari rings
- 1 tablespoon balsamic vinegar
- ½ tablespoon soy sauce
- 1 tablespoon sugar
- 1 cup veggie stock
- ½ teaspoon turmeric powder
- ½ teaspoon sweet paprika
- ½ cup chicken stock

Directions:

1. In your slow cooker, mix the calamari rings with the vinegar, soy sauce, and the other fixing, toss, put the

lid on and cook on high for 6 hours. Divide into bowls and serve right away as an appetizer.

Nutrition:

Calories: 230

Fat: 2g

Carbs: 7g

Protein: 5g

Chicken Bites

Preparation time: 15 minutes

Cooking time: 7 hours

Servings: 4 people

Ingredients:

- 1-pound chicken thighs, boneless and skinless
- 1 tbsp ginger, grated
- 1 yellow onion, sliced
- 1 tbsp garlic, minced
- 2 tsp cumin, ground
- 1 tsp cinnamon powder
- 2 tbsp sweet paprika
- 1 & ½ cups chicken stock
- 2 tbsp lemon juice
- ½ cup green olives pitted and roughly chopped

- Salt

- 3 tbsp olive oil

- 5 pita bread, cut in quarters and warmed in the oven

Directions:

1. Heat-up a pan with the olive oil over medium-high heat, put onions, garlic, ginger, salt, and pepper, stir and cook for 2 minutes. Put the cumin and cinnamon, mix well, and take off the heat.

2. Put chicken pieces in your slow cooker, then the onions mix, lemon juice, olives plus stock, stir, cover and cook on low within 7 hours. Shred meat, stir the whole mixture again, divide it on pita chips, and serve as a snack.

Nutrition: Calories: 265 Fat: 7g Carbs: 14g Protein: 6g

Maple Glazed Turkey Strips

Preparation time: 15 minutes

Cooking time: 3 hours & 30 minutes

Servings: 4 people

Ingredients:

- 15 oz. turkey fillets, cut into strips
- 2 tbsp honey
- 1 tbsp maple syrup
- 1 tsp cayenne pepper
- 1 tbsp butter
- 1 tsp paprika
- 1 tsp oregano
- 1 tsp dried dill
- 2 tbsp mayo

Directions:

1. Place the turkey strips in the slow cooker. Add all other spices, herbs, and mayo on top of the turkey.

2. Put the cooker's lid on and set the cooking time to 3 hours on high. During this time, mix honey with maple syrup and melted butter in a bowl.

3. Pour this honey glaze over the turkey evenly. Put the cooker's lid on and set the cooking time to 30 minutes on high. Serve warm.

Nutrition:

Calories: 295

Fat: 25.2g

Carbs: 6.82g

Protein: 10g

Lentils Rolls

Preparation time: 15 minutes

Cooking time: 8 hours

Servings: 4 people

Ingredients:

- 1 cup brown lentils, cooked
- 1 green cabbage head, leaves separated
- ½ cup onion, chopped
- 1 cup brown rice, already cooked
- 2 oz. white mushrooms, chopped
- ¼ cup pine nuts, toasted
- ¼ cup raisins
- 2 garlic cloves, minced
- 2 tablespoons dill, chopped
- 1 tablespoon olive oil

- 25 oz. marinara sauce

- A pinch of salt and black pepper

- ¼ cup of water

Directions:

1. In a bowl, mix lentils with onion, rice, mushrooms, pine nuts, raisins, garlic, dill, salt, and pepper, and whisk well.

2. Arrange cabbage leaves on a working surface, divide lentils mix and wrap them well. Add marinara sauce and water to your slow cooker and stir.

3. Add cabbage rolls, cover, and cook on low for 8 hours. Arrange cabbage rolls on a platter and serve.

Nutrition: Calories: 281, Fat: 6g, Carbs: 12g, Protein: 3g

Cauliflower Bites

Preparation time: 15 minutes

Cooking time: 4 hours

Servings: 2 people

Ingredients:

- 2 cups cauliflower florets
- 1 tablespoon Italian seasoning
- 1 tablespoon sweet paprika
- 2 tablespoons tomato sauce
- 1 teaspoon sweet paprika
- 1 tablespoon olive oil
- ¼ cup veggie stock

Directions:

1. In your slow cooker, mix the cauliflower florets with the Italian seasoning and the other fixing, toss, cook on low within 4 hours. Serve.

Nutrition:

Calories: 251

Fat: 4g

Carbs: 7g

Protein: 3g

Lemon Peel Snack

Preparation time: 15 minutes

Cooking time: 4 hours

Servings: 4 people

Ingredients:

- 5 big lemons, sliced halves, pulp removed and peel cut into strips
- 2 and ¼ cups white sugar
- 5 cups of water

Directions:

1. Put strips in your slow cooker, add water and sugar, stir cover and cook on low for 4 hours. Drain lemon peel and keep in jars until serving.

Nutrition: Calories: 7, Fat: 1g, Carbs: 2g, Protein: 1g

Peanut Snack

Preparation time: 10 minutes

Cooking time: 1 hour and 30 minutes

Servings: 4 people

Ingredients:

- 1 cup peanuts

- 1 cup chocolate peanut butter

- 12 oz. dark chocolate chips

- 12 oz. white chocolate chips

Directions:

1. In your slow cooker, mix peanuts with peanut butter, dark and white chocolate chips, cook on low within 1 hour and 30 minutes. Divide this mix into small muffin cups, leave aside to cool down, and serve as a snack.

Nutrition: Calories: 200, Fat: 4g, Carbs: 10g, Protein: 5g

Zucchini & Spinach with Bacon

Preparation time: 10 minutes

Cooking time: 6 hours

Servings: 4 people

Ingredients:

- 8 slices bacon

- 1 tablespoon olive oil

- 4 medium zucchinis, cubed

- 2 cups baby spinach

- 1 red onion, diced

- 6 garlic cloves, sliced thin

- 1 cup chicken broth

- salt and pepper to taste

Directions:

1. Warm-up olive oil in a pan, brown the bacon for 5 minutes. Break it into pieces in the pan. Place remaining ingredients in the slow cooker, pour the bacon and fat from the pan over the fixing inside the slow cooker. Cover, cook on low for 6 hours.

Nutrition:

Calories: 290, Carbs: 16g, Fat: 20g, Protein: 12g

Pepperoni Pizza with Meat Crust

Preparation time: 5 minutes

Cooking time: 4 hours

Servings: 4 people

Ingredients:

- 2.2. pounds lean ground beef

- 2 garlic cloves, minced

- 1 tablespoon dry, fried onions

- salt and pepper to taste

- 2 cups shredded mozzarella

- 1 ¾ cup sugarless ready-made pizza sauce

- 2 cups shredded yellow cheese, cheddar

- ½ cup sliced pepperoni

Directions:

1. Brown the beef with the seasoning in a pan. Mix the beef with the cheese. Butter the slow cooker and spread the crust out evenly over the bottom.

2. Pour the pizza sauce over the crust and spread evenly. Top with the cheese and arrange the pepperoni slices. Cover, cook on low for 4 hours. Serve.

Nutrition:

Calories: 320, Carbs: 31g, Fat: 16g, Protein: 15g

Spinach & Sausage Pizza

Preparation time: 5 minutes

Cooking time: 6 hours

Servings: 4 people

Ingredients:

- 1 tablespoon olive oil

- 1 cup lean ground beef

- 2 cups spicy pork sausage

- 2 garlic cloves, minced

- 1 tablespoon dry, fried onions

- salt and pepper to taste

- 1 ¾ cups sugarless ready-made pizza sauce

- 3 cups fresh spinach

- ½ cup sliced pepperoni

- ¼ cup pitted black olives, sliced

- ¼ cup sun-dried tomatoes, chopped

- ½ cup spring onions, chopped

- 3 cups shredded mozzarella

Directions:

1. In a pan, heat the olive oil. Brown the beef, then the pork. Drain the oil off the meat, then mix. Pour the meat into the slow cooker.

2. Spread evenly and press down. Alternate in layers the pizza sauce, toppings, and cheese. Cover and cook on low within 4-6 hours. Serve.

Nutrition:

Calories: 314, Carbs: 34g, Fat: 12g, Protein: 17g

Greek-Style Frittata with

Spinach and Feta Cheese

Preparation time: 10 minutes

Cooking time: 4 hours

Servings: 4 people

Ingredients:

- 2 cups spinach, fresh or frozen

- 8 eggs, lightly beaten

- 1 cup plain yogurt

- 1 small onion, cut into small pieces

- 2 red roasted peppers, peeled

- 1 garlic clove, crushed

- 1 cup feta cheese, crumbled

- 2 tablespoons softened butter

- 2 tablespoons olive oil

- salt and pepper to taste

- 1 teaspoon dried oregano

Directions:

1. Sauté the onion and garlic for 5 minutes. Add the spinach, heat for an additional 2 minutes. Let the mixture cool down.

2. Roast the red peppers in a dry pan or under the broiler. Peel them and cut them into small pieces.

3. Beat the eggs, yogurt, and seasoning in a separate bowl. Combine well. Add the peppers and the onion mixture. Mix again.

4. Crumble the feta cheese using a fork, add it to the frittata. Grease the bottom and sides of the slow cooker with butter. Pour the mixture into it. Cover, cook on low for 4 hours.

Nutrition: Calories: 206 Carbs: 13g Fat: 13g Protein: 11g

Nut & Zucchini Bread

Preparation time: 10 minutes

Cooking time: 3 hours

Servings: 4 people

Ingredients:

- 2 cups shredded zucchini

- ½ cup ground walnuts

- 1 cup ground almonds

- 1/3 cup coconut flakes

- 2 teaspoons cinnamon

- ½ teaspoon baking soda

- 1 ½ teaspoons baking powder

- ½ teaspoon salt

- 3 large eggs

- 1/3 cup softened coconut oil

- 1 cup sweetener, Swerve (or a suitable substitute)

- 2 teaspoons vanilla

Directions:

1. Shred the zucchini and ground the walnuts. In a bowl, beat the eggs, oil, sweetener, and vanilla together.

2. Add the dry ingredients to the wet mixture. Fold in the zucchini and walnuts. Pour the batter into your bread pan, which fits inside the slow cooker.

3. Crumble aluminum foil into four balls, place on the bottom of the slow cooker, and set the pan in the slow cooker with a paper towel on top to absorb the water—cook on high for 3 hours. Cool, wrap in foil, and refrigerate. Serve cold with tea or coffee.

Nutrition: Calories: 90, Carbs: 12g, Fat: 4g, Protein: 1g

Cheese & Cauliflower Bake

Preparation time: 5 minutes

Cooking time: 4 hours

Servings: 4 people

Ingredients:

- 1 head cauliflower, cut into florets

- ½ cup cream cheese

- ¼ cup whipping cream

- 2 tablespoons lard or butter

- 1 tablespoon lard or butter to grease the slow cooker

- 1 teaspoon salt

- ½ teaspoon fresh ground black pepper

- ½ cup yellow cheese, cheddar, shredded

- 6 slices of bacon, crisped and crumbled

Directions:

1. Grease the slow cooker. Add all the fixing, except the cheese and the bacon. Cook on low for 3 hours. Open the lid and add cheese. Re-cover, cook for an additional hour. Top with the bacon and serve.

Tip: Good for brunch with a couple of cherry tomatoes and avocado slices.

Nutrition:

Calories: 178, Carbs: 8g, Fat: 11g, Protein: 5g

Ham & Cheese Broccoli Brunch

Bowl

Preparation time: 5 minutes

Cooking time: 8 hours

Servings: 4 people

Ingredients:

- 1 medium head of broccoli, chopped small

- 4 cups vegetable broth

- 2 tablespoons olive oil

- 1 teaspoon mustard seeds, ground

- 3 garlic cloves, minced

- salt and pepper to taste

- 2 cups cheddar cheese, shredded

- 2 cups ham, cubed

- pinch of paprika

Directions:

1. Add all ingredients to the 6-quart slow cooker in order of the list. Cover, cook on low for 8 hours.

Nutrition: Calories: 320

Carbs: 28g

Fat: 17g

Protein: 14g

Eggplant & Sausage Bake

Preparation time: 10 minutes

Cooking time: 4 hours

Servings: 4 people

Ingredients:

- 2 cups eggplant, cubed, salted, and drained

- 1 tablespoon olive oil

- 2 pounds spicy pork sausage

- 1 tablespoon Worcestershire sauce

- 1 tablespoon mustard

- 2 regular cans Italian diced tomatoes

- 1 jar tomato passata

- 2 cups mozzarella cheese, shredded

Directions:

1. Grease the slow cooker with olive oil. Mix the sausage, Worcestershire sauce, and mustard. Pour the mixture into the slow cooker.

2. Top the meat mixture with eggplant. Pour the tomatoes over the batter, sprinkle with grated cheese. Cover, cook on low for 4 hours. Enjoy for brunch.

Nutrition: Calories: 345

Carbs: 34g

Fat: 15g

Protein: 21g

Three-Cheese Artichoke Hearts Bake

Preparation time: 5 minutes

Cooking time: 2 hours

Servings: 4 people

Ingredients:

- 1 cup cheddar cheese, grated

- ½ cup dry parmesan cheese

- 1 cup cream cheese

- 1 cup spinach, chopped

- 1 clove of garlic, crushed

- 1 jar artichoke hearts, chopped

- salt and pepper to taste

Directions:

1. Place all the ingredients in the 6-quart slow cooker. Mix lightly. Cover, cook on high for 2 hours. Serve.

Nutrition:

Calories: 40

Carbs: 7g

Fat: 0g

Protein: 2g

Sweet Ham Maple Breakfast

Preparation time: 15 minutes

Cooking time: 3-4 hours

Servings: 4 people

Ingredients:

- 3-pound fully-cooked boneless ham

- ½ cup of maple syrup

- ½ cup of Honey Dijon Mustard

- ½ cup of packed brown sugar

Directions:

1. Make cross-shaped diagonal patterns on the ham with a knife and place them into a slow cooker. In a

large bowl, whisk together the rest of the ingredients and pour over the ham.

2. Cover and cook on low within 3-4 hours. Take the ham out and cover with foil for 10 minutes. Slice and serve.

Nutrition: Calories: 430

Fat: 24g

Protein: 32g,

Carbs: 13g

Sausage Casserole Breakfast

Preparation time: 15 minutes

Cooking time: 4-5 hours

Servings: 4 people

Ingredients:

- 8 large eggs

- 1 ½ cups of low-fat milk

- 1 pound of cooked bulk sausage, drained

- 1 seeded and chopped jalapeño

- 1 chopped red bell pepper

- ¾ cup sliced green onions

- 2 cups of low-fat Mexican blend cheese

- 9 corn tortillas

- ½ cup of salsa

Directions:

1. Mix the eggs, jalapeño, and milk in a large bowl. In another large bowl, combine the cheese, green onions, sausage, and red bell pepper.

2. Arrange 3 tortillas on the base of a greased slow cooker. Spread a layer of the sausage mixture over the tortillas.

3. Repeat the layering, and then pour the egg mixture over the top. Cover and cook on low within 4-5 hours. Divide onto plates and serve with the salsa.

Nutrition: Calories: 386 Fat: 24g Fiber: 2.6g Protein: 24.7g

Mushroom Bacon Breakfast

Preparation time: 15 minutes

Cooking time: 4-6 hours

Servings: 4 people

Ingredients:

- 2 cups of ground sausage, cooked

- ½ cup of chopped onion

- 1 tablespoon of dried parsley

- 1 teaspoon of garlic powder

- 1 teaspoon of thyme

- 6 slices of bacon, cooked and crumbled

- 2 cups of organic chicken broth

- 1 red bell pepper, chopped

- ½ cup of parmesan cheese

- 1 cup of heavy cream

- 2 cups of sliced mushrooms

- Salt and black pepper

Directions:

1. Place all of the fixings into a large slow cooker. Cook within 4-6 hours on a low setting.

2. Ensure that you don't overcook the ingredients or cook the food at too high heat. It will cause the cream to separate. When the food is cooked, divide onto plates and serve hot.

Nutrition:

Calories: 166, Carbs: 2.1g, Fat: 15.5g, Fiber: 0.3g, Protein:6.7g

Zucchini Cinnamon Nut Bread

Preparation time: 15 minutes

Cooking time: 3 hours

Servings: 4 people

Ingredients:

- 2 cups of zucchini, shredded

- ½ cup of ground walnuts

- 1 cup of ground almonds

- 1/3 cup of coconut flakes

- 2 teaspoons of cinnamon

- ½ teaspoon of baking soda

- 1 ½ teaspoon of baking powder

- ½ teaspoon of salt

- 3 large eggs

- 1/3 cup of softened coconut oil

- 1 cup of sweetener of your choice

- 2 teaspoons of vanilla

Directions:

1. In a large bowl, beat the vanilla, sweetener, oil, and eggs and whisk them together thoroughly. Add all of the dry fixings to the egg mixture. Add the walnuts and the zucchini.

2. You will need a bread pan that is small enough to fit into the slow cooker. Pour the batter into it. Roll up aluminum foil into four balls and set them on the base of the slow cooker.

3. Put the pan into your slow cooker and place a paper towel over the top to absorb condensation. Cook on high for 3 hours.

4. Allow the bread to cool down, wrap it in foil and place it in the fridge. Serve cold with coffee or tea.

Nutrition:

Calories: 210

Carbs: 4g

Protein: 5g

Fat: 18g

Ham and Spinach Frittata

Preparation time: 15 minutes

Cooking time: 2 hours

Servings: 4 people

Ingredients:

- 10 large eggs

- ½ diced green bell pepper, diced

- 1 cup of ham, diced

- 2 handfuls of fresh spinach

- Salt and pepper

Directions:

1. Put a parchment liner in your slow cooker and grease it with non-stick cooking spray. Put the peppers, spinach, and ham into the slow cooker.

2. Whisk the eggs into your large bowl. Add salt and pepper, and then pour the eggs into the slow cooker.

3. Cook the ingredients on high for 1 ½ to 2 hours. Slice the frittata, divide onto plates, and serve.

Nutrition:

Calories: 109

Fat: 6.9g

Carbs: 1.8g

Protein: 5.6g

Cheese Grits

Preparation time: 5 minutes

Cooking time: 5-7 hours

Servings: 4 people

Ingredients:

- 1/2 cup stone-ground grits

- 5-6 cups of water

- 2 tsp salt

- 1/2 cup Cheddar cheese (shredded)

- 6 tbsp butter

- Black pepper (optionally)

Directions:

1. Preheat slow cooker on low, spray the dish with cooking spray, or cover with butter. In a wide bowl, mix grits and water, add salt. Cook on low temperatures for 5-7 hours; you can leave it overnight.

2. Remove the dish from the slow cooker, cover butter on top. Stir with the whisk to an even consistency and fully melted butter.

3. To serve, sprinkle more cheese on top and black pepper to your taste. Serve warm.

Nutrition:

Calories: 173

Fat: 7g

Carbs: 4g

Protein: 6g

Pineapple Cake with Pecans

Preparation time: 15 minutes

Cooking time: 3-4 hours

Servings: 4 people

Ingredients:

- 2 cups of sugar

- 2 cups plain flour

- 2 eggs

- 4 tbsp vegetable oil

- 1 can pineapple with juice (crushed)

- 1 tsp baking soda

- 1 tsp vanilla extract

- Salt

For icing:

- 1 cup of sugar

- 1/2 cup butter

- 6 tbsp evaporated milk

- 3 tbsp shredded coconut

- 1/2 cup chopped pecans (toasted)

Directions:

1. Preheat your slow cooker to 180-200°F. Take a medium bowl and combine all cake ingredients.

2. Mix the dough until evenly combined and then pour into slow cooker dish. Bake for 3 hours on high; check if it is ready with a wooden toothpick.

3. When the cake is ready, make the icing: in a medium saucepan, combine sugar, evaporated milk, butter, and salt. Bring to boil; and then simmer with a lower heat for 10 minutes.

4. Add the coconut to the icing. Put the icing over the hot cake, then sprinkle with nuts. To serve, let the cake cool, then cut it and serve with your favorite drinks.

Nutrition:

Calories: 291

Fat: 7g

Carbs: 6g

Protein: 5g

Potato Casserole for Breakfast

Preparation time: 5 minutes

Cooking time: 4 hours

Servings: 4 people

Ingredients:

- 4 big potatoes

- 5-6 sausages

- 1/2 cup cheddar cheese (shredded)

- 1/2 cup mozzarella cheese

- 5-6 green onions

- 10 chicken eggs

- 1/2 cup milk

- Salt

- Black pepper

Directions:

1. Preheat slow cooker on low; spray its dish with non-stick cooking spray. Rub the potatoes into small pieces and put them into the dish.

2. Cover the potatoes with rubbed sausages. Add both mozzarella, cheddar cheeses, and green onions. Continue the layers until all space in the dish is full.

3. Mix the wet ingredients (milk, eggs) in a medium bowl. Pour it into the main dish, then put salt and pepper. Leave to cook on low for 5 hours or until the eggs are set. Serve with guacamole or green onions.

Nutrition:

Calories: 190, Fat: 10g, Carbs: 5g, Protein: 10g

Cinnamon Rolls

Preparation time: 15 minutes

Cooking time: 2 hours

Servings: 10-12 pieces

Ingredients:

- 2 cups warm water

- 1 tbsp active yeast (dry)

- 2 tbsp wild honey

- 3 cups plain flour

- 1 tsp salt

- 4 tbsp butter

- 4 tbsp brown sugar

- 1 tsp cinnamon

Directions:

1. In a bowl, mix up water, yeast, and honey. Stir with a mixer and after the dough is homogenous, let it rest for several minutes; mixture will rise.

2. Sift flour and add salt. Mix on low to let the ingredients come together, then increase the mixing speed to medium. Remove dough and allow to rise on a floured table.

3. Roll dough into medium rectangles. You can use a pizza cutter to make the sides even. Spread the butter over the dough. Sprinkle it with sugar and cinnamon.

4. Roll the dough rectangles into a long log, and then cut it into 10-12 pieces. Cover your slow cooker inside with foil, place the rolls over it and cook on high for 2-3 hours. To serve, use fresh berries or mint leaves.

Nutrition:

Calories: 190, Fat: 5g, Carbs: 7g, Protein: 8g

Quinoa Pie

Preparation time: 10 minutes

Cooking time: 4 hours

Servings: 4 people

Ingredients:

- 2 tbsp almond butter

- 2 tbsp maple syrup

- 1 cup vanilla almond milk

- 1 tsp salt

- 1/2 cup quinoa

- 2 chicken eggs

- Cinnamon

- 1/2 cup raisins

- 5 tbsp roasted almonds (chopped)

- 1/2 cup dried apples

Directions:

1. Spray the slow cooker dish with no-stick spray or cover it with foil or parchment paper. In another bowl, mix the almond butter and maple syrup. Melt in a microwave until creamy, about a minute.

2. Add almond milk, salt, and cinnamon, then whisk the mass until it is entirely even. Add the eggs and remaining products, mix well. Preheat your slow cooker to 100-110°F.

3. Put the dough into the dish, then place it into the slow cooker. Cook for 3-4 hours on high. To serve, remove the pie out of the dish with a knife. Cool in the refrigerator.

Nutrition: Calories: 174,, Fat: 8g, Carbs: 20g, Protein: 6g

Quinoa Muffins with Peanut Butter

Preparation time: 10 minutes

Cooking time: 4 hours

Servings: 8 muffins

Ingredients:

- 1 cup strawberries

- 1/2 cup almond vanilla milk

- 1 tsp salt

- 5-6 tbsp raw quinoa

- 2 tbsp peanut butter (better natural)

- 3 tbsp honey

- 4 egg whites

- 2 tbsp peanuts (roasted)

Directions:

1. Preheat your slow cooker to 190°F. Line the cooking dish bottom with parchment paper; additionally, spray it with cooking spray. Dice the strawberries and place them over the dish.

2. Sprinkle with honey and place the dish into the slow cooker for 10-15 minutes for releasing juices. In another pot, mix up the almond milk and salt. Boil with quinoa until ready.

3. Combine egg whites and almond butter in a separate bowl. Put the quinoa and wait until milk is absorbed.

4. Fill the muffin forms with quinoa mixture; place the strawberries on the top. Bake in the slow cooker on low until quinoa is set for about 4 hours. To serve, cool the muffins and decorate them with whole strawberries.

Nutrition: Calories: 190, Fat: 6g, Carbs: 8g, Protein: 6g

Veggie Omelets

Preparation time: 5 minutes

Cooking time: 2 hours

Servings: 8 pieces

Ingredients:

- 6 chicken eggs

- 1/2 cup milk

- salt

- garlic powder

- white pepper

- red pepper

- small onion

- garlic clove

- parsley

- 5 small tomatoes

Directions:

1. Grease the slow cooker dish with butter or special cooking spray. In a separate bowl, mix up eggs and milk. Add pepper and garlic.

2. Whisk the mixture well and salt. Add to the mixture broccoli florets, onions, pepper, and garlic. Stir in the eggs.

3. Place the mixture into the slow cooker dish. Cook on high temperatures at 180-200°F for 2 hours. Cover with cheese and let it melt. To serve, cut the omelet into 8 pieces and garnish the plates with parsley and tomatoes.

Nutrition: Calories: 210, Fat: 7g, Carbs: 5g, Protein: 8g

Apple Pie with Oatmeal

Preparation time: 10 minutes

Cooking time: 4-6 hours

Servings: 4 people

Ingredients:

- 1 cup oats

- 2 large apples

- 2 cups almond milk

- 2 cups warm water

- 2 tsp cinnamon

- Pinch nutmeg

- Salt

- 2 tbsp coconut oil

- 1 tsp vanilla extract

- 2 tbsp flaxseeds

- 2 tbsp maple syrup

- Raisins

Directions:

1. Grease your slow cooker. Rub a couple of spoons of coconut or olive oil. Peel the apples. Core and chop them into medium size pieces.

2. Starting with the apples, add all the ingredients into the slow cooker. Stir and leave to bake for 6 hours on low. When ready, stir the oatmeal well.

3. Serve the oatmeal into small cups. You can also garnish it with any berries or toppings you like.

Nutrition: Calories: 159, Fat: 12g, Carbs: 9g, Protein: 28g

Vanilla French Toast

Preparation time: 15 minutes

Cooking time: 8 hours/overnight

Servings: 4 people

Ingredients:

- 1 loaf bread (better day-old)

- 2 cups cream

- 2 cups milk, whole

- 8 eggs

- almond extract

- 1 vanilla bean

- 5 tsp sugar

- Cinnamon

- Salt

Directions:

1. Coat the slow cooker dish with the cooking spray. Slice bread into small pieces (1-2 inches). Place them into the dish overlapping each other. In another dish, combine the remaining ingredients until perfectly blended.

2. Pour the wet mixture over the bread to cover it completely. Place the dish into a slow cooker and cook on low at 100-120°F for 7-8 hours. To serve, slightly cool and cut the French toast.

Nutrition:

Calories: 200, Fat: 6g

Carbs: 4g

Protein: 8g

Greek Eggs Casserole

Preparation time: 15 minutes

Cooking time: 6 hours

Servings: 4 people

Ingredients:

- 10 chicken eggs

- 1/2 cup milk

- Salt

- 1 tsp black pepper

- 1 tbsp red onion

- 1/2 cup dried tomatoes

- 1 cup champignons

- 2cups spinach

- 1/2 cup feta

Directions:

1. Set your slow cooker to 120-150°F. In a separate wide bowl, combine and whisk the eggs. Add salt and pepper. Mix in garlic and red onion. Whisk again.

2. Wash and dice the mushrooms. Put them into the wet mixture. At last, and add dried tomatoes. Pour the mixture into the slow cooker.

3. Top the meal with the feta cheese and cook on low for 5-6 hours. Serve with milk or vegetables.

Nutrition:

Calories: 180

Fat: 8g

Carbs: 4g

Protein: 8g

Banana Bread

Preparation time: 15 minutes

Cooking time: 4 hours

Servings: 3 people

Ingredients:

- 2 chicken eggs

- 1/2 cup softened butter

- 1 cup of sugar

- 2 cups plain flour

- 1/2 teaspoon baking soda

- Salt

- 3 medium bananas

Directions:

1. First, cover with cooking spray and preheat your slow cooker. Combine eggs with sugar and butter. Stir well. Mix in baking soda and baking powder.

2. Peel and mash bananas, mix them with flour, and combine with eggs. Pour the dough into the cooking dish and place it into the slow cooker. Cook on low for 3-4 hours.

3. When ready, remove the bread with a knife and enjoy your breakfast! To serve, use fresh bananas, apples, or berries to your taste.

Nutrition:

Calories: 130

Fat: 8g

Carbs: 5g

Protein: 7g

www.ingramcontent.com/pod-product-compliance
Lightning Source LLC
Chambersburg PA
CBHW071111030426
42336CB00013BA/2037